I HAD A **BLACK** DOG

HIS NAME WAS DEPRESSION

PRAISE FOR *I HAD A BLACK DOG*

'What a fascinating book. It is both instructive and accessible. I am sure it will have a universal appeal.'
Dr Rosemary Leonard, resident medical adviser for BBC1's *Breakfast*

'I found it a moving and surprisingly funny insight into depression and how to find hope in darkness. I didn't think "self-help" and "picture book" were two genres that could be fruitfully combined, but Matthew Johnstone blends them into something genuinely inspiring.'
Oliver Burkeman, *Guardian*

'It's very accurate — I should know!'
Ruby Wax

'Describing the hell of depression to other people, even those who really want to help, can be so daunting that sufferers find it impossible to reach out. Matthew Johnstone's cartoon book about confronting and ultimately befriending his own black dog cuts through the taboos in a simple, effective and touching way.'
Sarah Stacey, Health Editor, *YOU magazine*

'Truthful, touching and hopeful'
Dr James Le Fanu, medical columnist, *Daily Telegraph*

'His highly original mix of genres — autobiographical/self-help in picture-book format proved just what the doctor ordered'
Spectrum, *Sydney Morning Herald*

'This brilliant, disarming book about depression is quick to read, clever and poignant'
Australian Financial Review

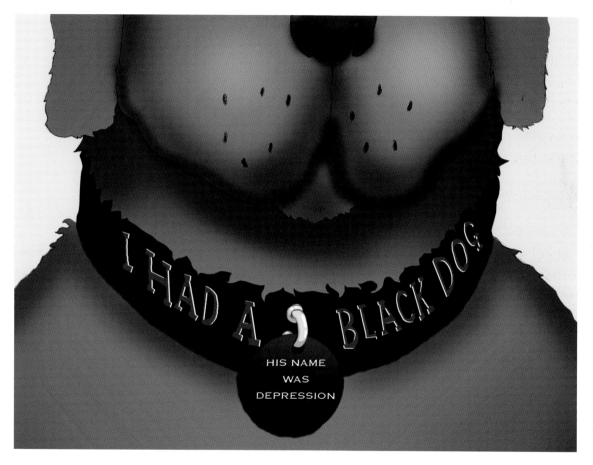

I HAD A BLACK DOG

HIS NAME
WAS
DEPRESSION

Written and illustrated by Matthew Johnstone

ROBINSON
London

(Not) for my family and friends

First published in Australia in 2005 by Pan, an imprint of Pan Macmillan Australia Pty Limited
St Martins Tower, 31 Market Street, Sydney

First published in Great Britain in 2007 by Robinson
an imprint of Constable & Robinson Ltd

9 10

A CIP catalogue record for this book
is available from the British Library.

ISBN 978-1-84529-589-9 (paperback)
ISBN 978-1-78033-903-0 (ebook)

Robinson
An imprint of
Little, Brown Book Group
Carmelite House
50 Victoria Embankment
London EC4Y 0DZ

An Hachette UK Company
www.hachette.co.uk

www.littlebrown.co.uk

Important Note
This book is not intended as a substitute for medical advice or treatment.
Any person with a condition requiring medical attention should consult
a qualified medical practitioner or suitable therapist.

FOREWORD

Depression comes in different guises and haunts the lives of many. Although 1 to 2 per cent of children can suffer depression, in most cases it begins with the onset of puberty. About 1 in 4 women and 1 in 7 to 8 men will have an episode of depression at some time in their lives, and women are twice as vulnerable as men.

Research has shown that during depression there are changes in certain chemicals in the brain and the way in which brain cells send signals to each other. When animals are subjected to various stresses over certain periods of time, we know that their brains change too and they can also appear depressed. Looked at this way, depression can be seen as a 'brain state' that once triggered will affect our thoughts, feelings and behaviours. Depression *is not* something to be ashamed about. There are in fact many ways to try to change these aspects of depression.

Matthew Johnstone takes us through his own personal experience of depression. He externalizes his depression by calling it 'Black Dog', a term that Winston Churchill also used. With these heart warming and insightful pictures Matthew reveals his journey. Matthew's touching observations can alight our own compassionate feelings for the state of depression, and through that help us to find new hope to bear and work through it.

The ability to see one's 'Black Dog' as something that is happening to you rather than the 'real you' can help you to think about your depression in a constructive manner. If you feel depressed, try to reach out to those who might be able to help you, including your family doctor. Helpful websites are also listed at the back of this book.

Paul Gilbert,
Professor of Clinical Psychology at the University of Derby and
Head of Specialty, Adult Mental Health for the Derbyshire Mental Health Trust

Looking back, Black Dog had been in and out
of my life since my early twenties.

Whenever he made an appearance, I felt empty
and life just seemed to slow down.

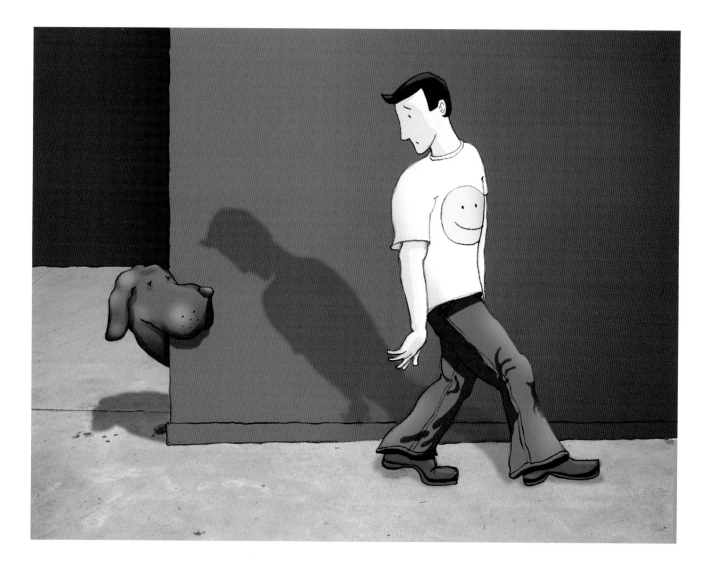

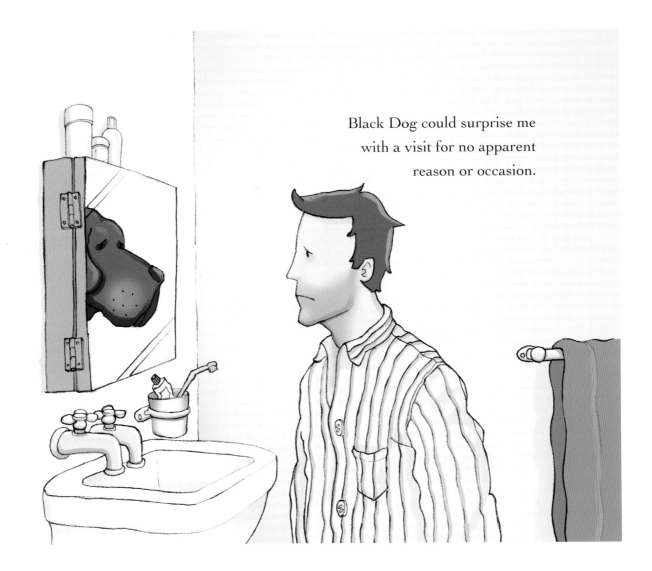

Black Dog could surprise me
with a visit for no apparent
reason or occasion.

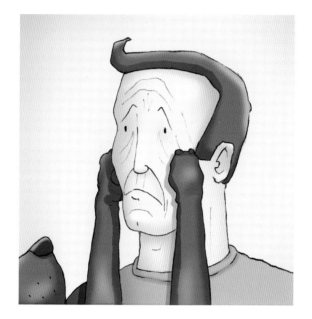

He could make me look and feel older than my years.

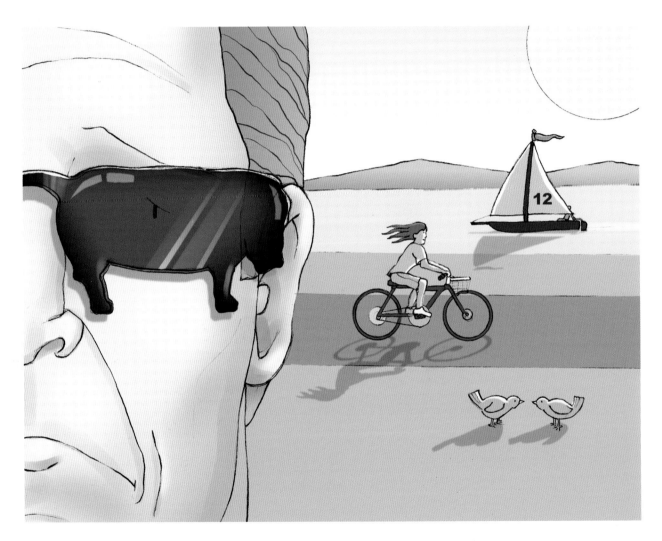

When the rest of the world seemed to be enjoying life, I could only see it through the Black Dog.

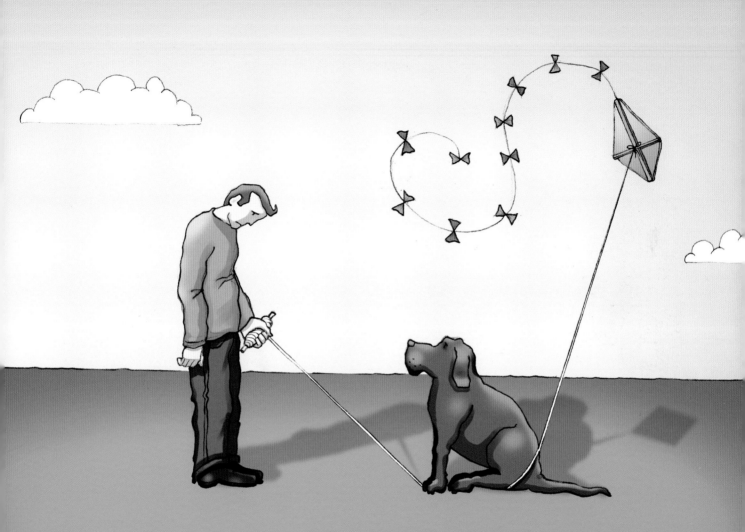

Activities that usually brought me pleasure suddenly ceased to.

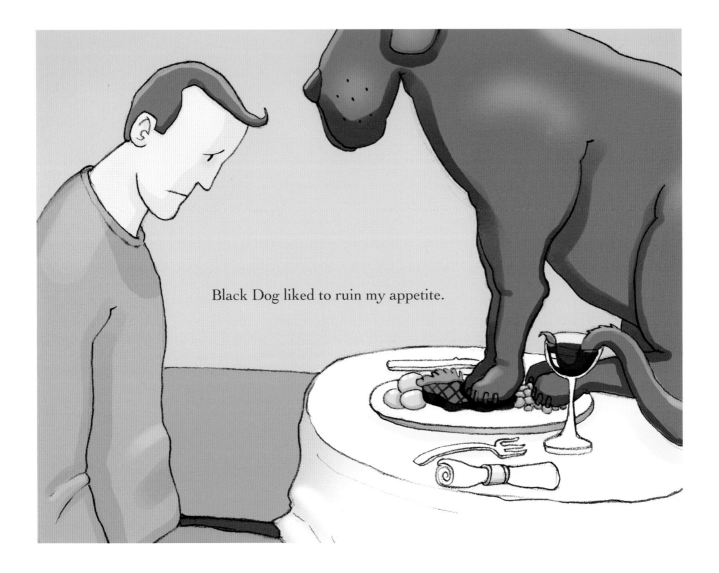

Black Dog liked to ruin my appetite.

He chewed up my memory and my ability to concentrate.

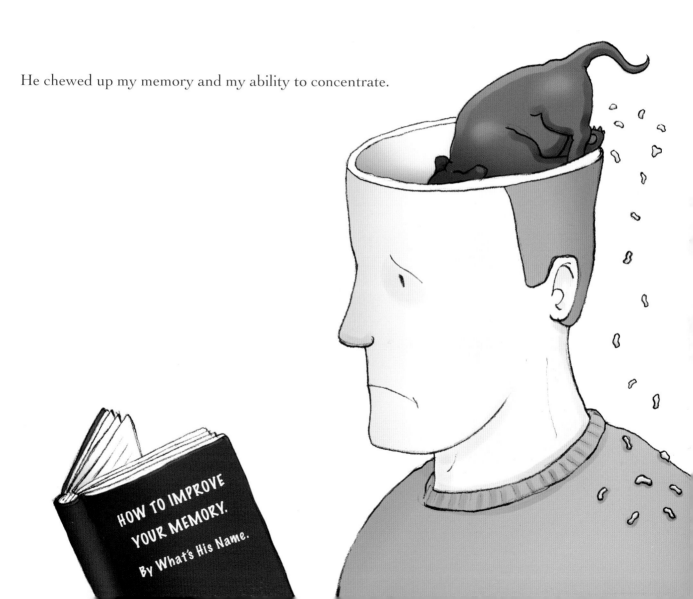

Doing anything or going anywhere with Black Dog
required superhuman strength.

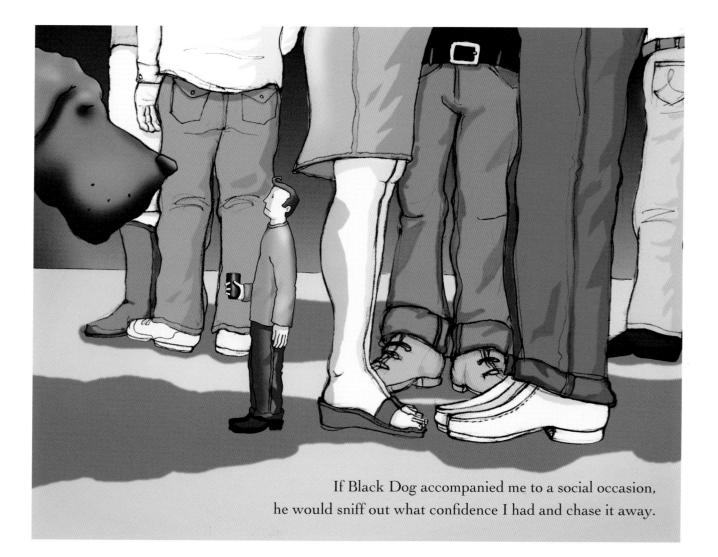

If Black Dog accompanied me to a social occasion,
he would sniff out what confidence I had and chase it away.

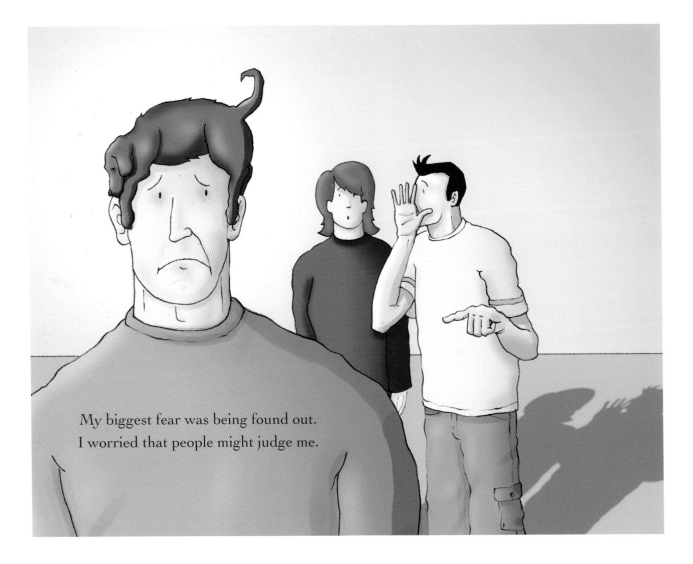

Because of the shame and stigma
associated with Black Dog,
I became a champion at fooling everyone,
both at home and at work.

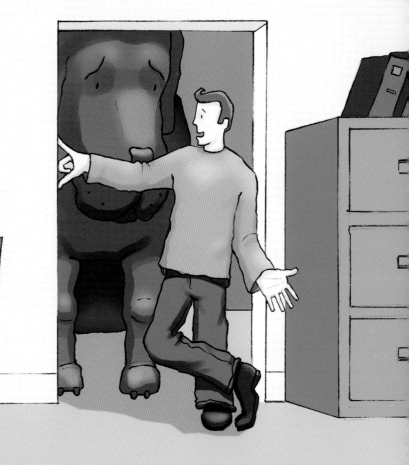

Keeping up an emotional lie takes an incredible amount of energy.
It's like trying to cover up epilepsy, a heart attack, or diabetes.

Black Dog could make me say negative things.

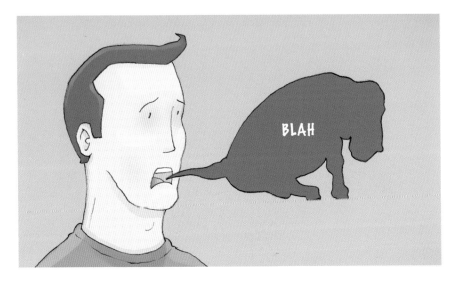

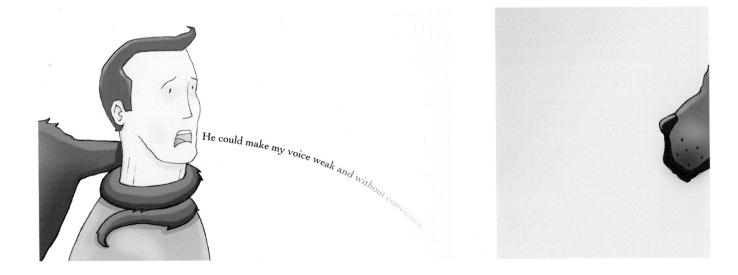

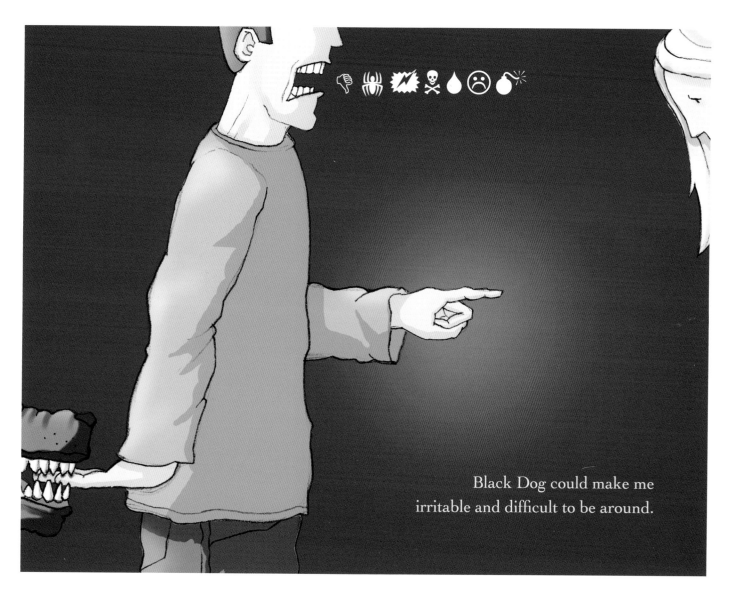

Black Dog could make me
irritable and difficult to be around.

Black Dog thought nothing of taking my love
and burying my intimacy.

3:20

He liked to wake me up with very repetitive, negative thinking.

Having a Black Dog in your life isn't so much

about feeling a bit down, sad or blue.

At its worst, it's about being devoid of feeling altogether.

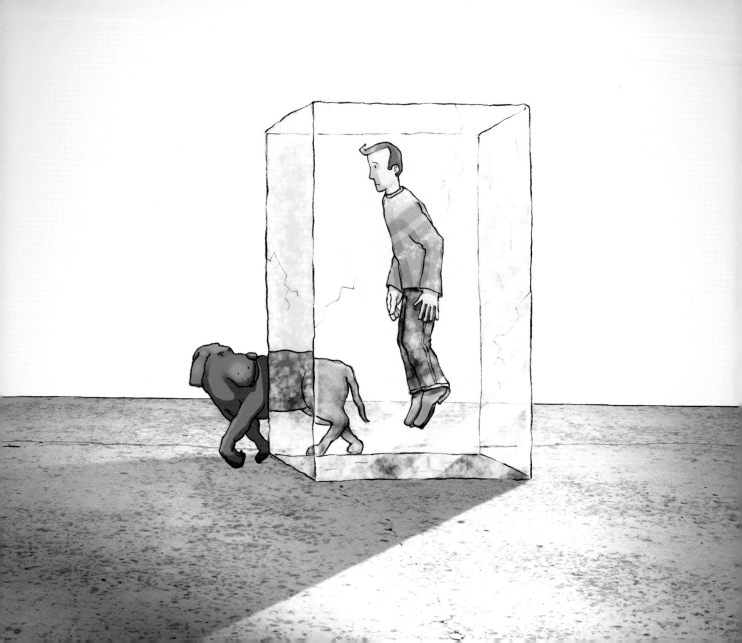

As the years went by, Black Dog got bigger and he started hanging around all the time.

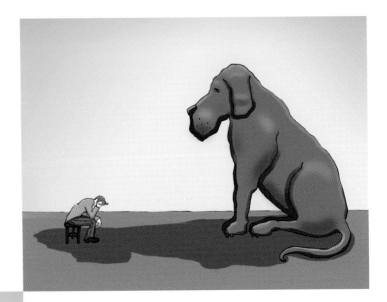

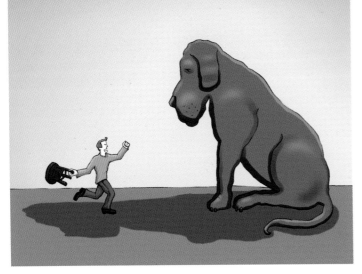

I would say THAT'S IT!!!
and attack him with whatever
I thought might send him running.

But more often than not, he would
come out on top. Going down became
easier than getting up again.

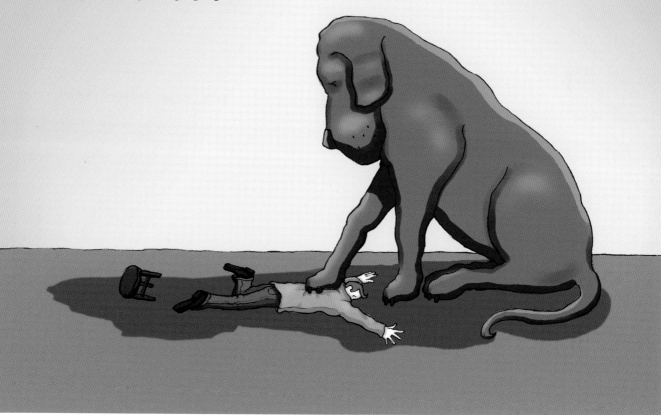

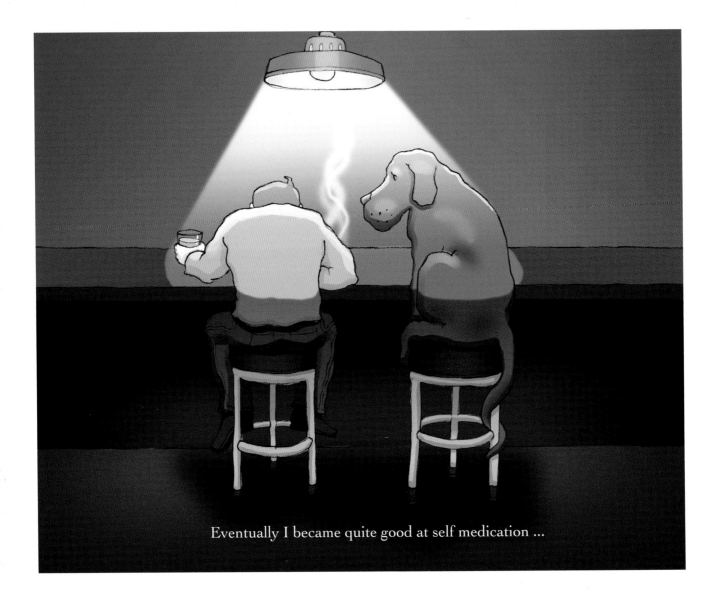

Eventually I became quite good at self medication ...

... which never really helped.

I began to feel totally isolated from everything and everyone.

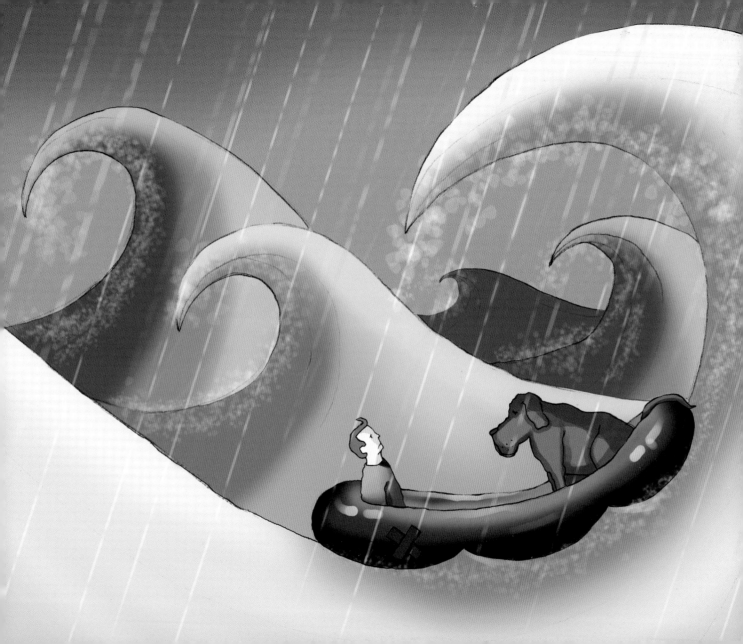

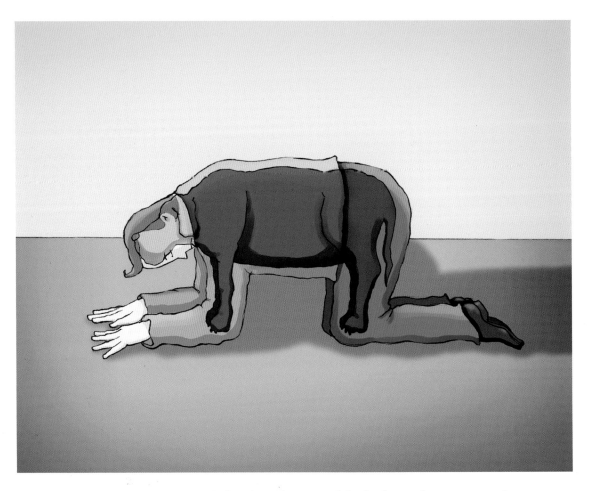

Black Dog finally succeeded in hijacking my life; he brought me to my knees.
My will to go on had deserted me.

Which was about the time I sought
professional help and got a clinical diagnosis.

This was my first step towards recovery and
was a major turning point in my life.

I discovered that there are many different breeds of Black Dog affecting millions of people from all walks of life. The Black Dog is an equal opportunity mongrel.

I learnt that there are many different ways to treat Black Dog. I also learnt that there is no quick fix.

Medication can be a necessary part of the treatment for some; others may need a different approach altogether.

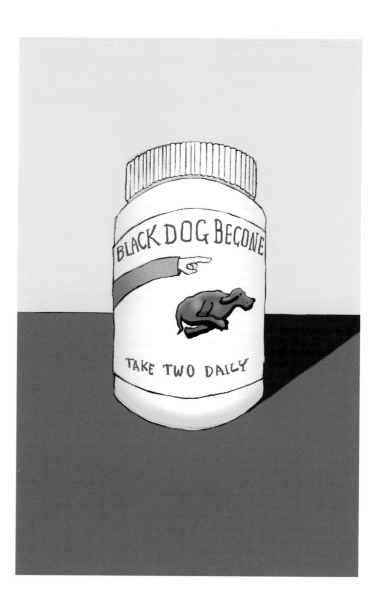

Black Dog had me believe that if I ever told anyone about him, I would be judged. The truth is, being emotionally genuine with close friends and family can be an absolute life saver.

BLACK DOGUS HORRIBILIS

Letting the Dog out is far better than keeping him in.

I learnt not to be afraid of Black Dog
and taught him a few tricks of my own.

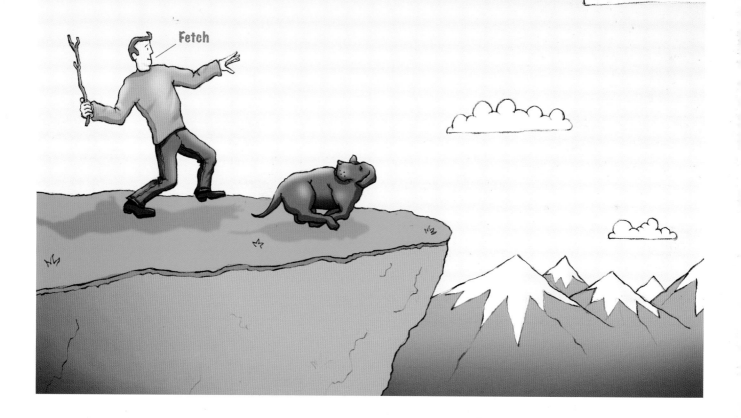

Black Dog feeds on stress and fatigue;
the more stressed you get the louder he barks.

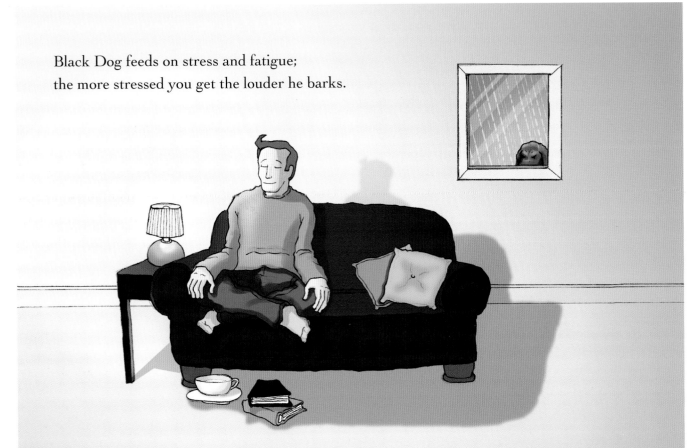

It's important to learn how to rest properly and quiet your mind.
Yoga, meditation and being in nature can help shut out the Dog.

Black Dog is fat and lazy, he would far rather you lie on your bed and feel sorry for yourself. He hates exercise mostly because it makes you feel better. When you least feel like moving is when you should move the most.

So go for a walk or run and leave the mutt behind.

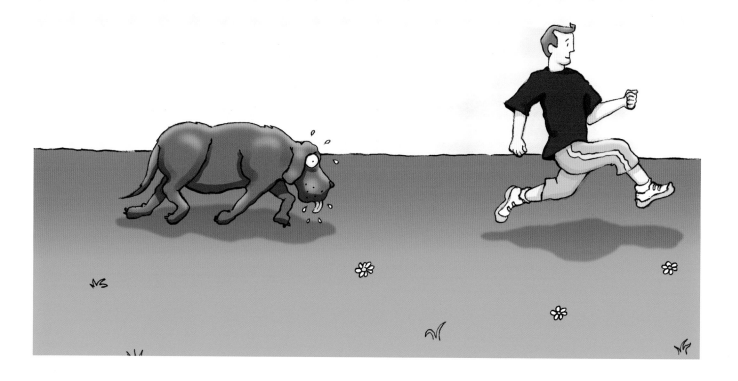

Keeping a mood journal can be very useful.
Getting your thoughts on paper
is highly liberating and often insightful.

Working out some sort of symbol for ranking
how you're feeling each day,
is a good way to keep track of the Dog.

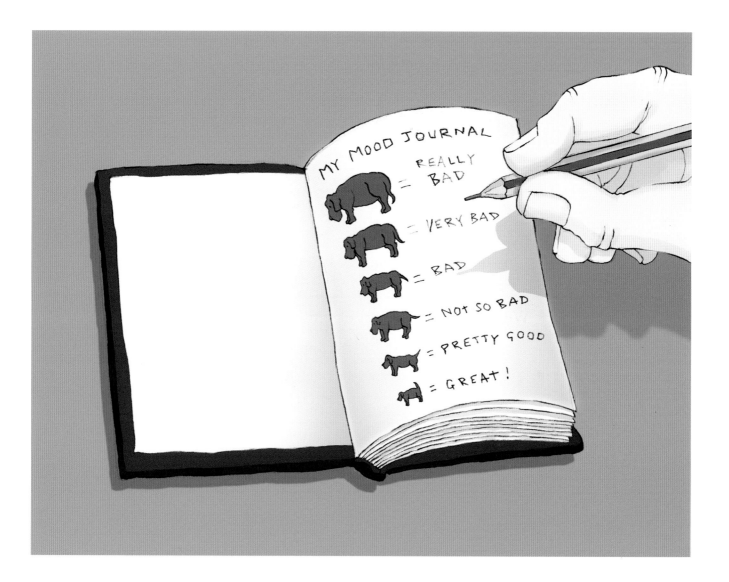

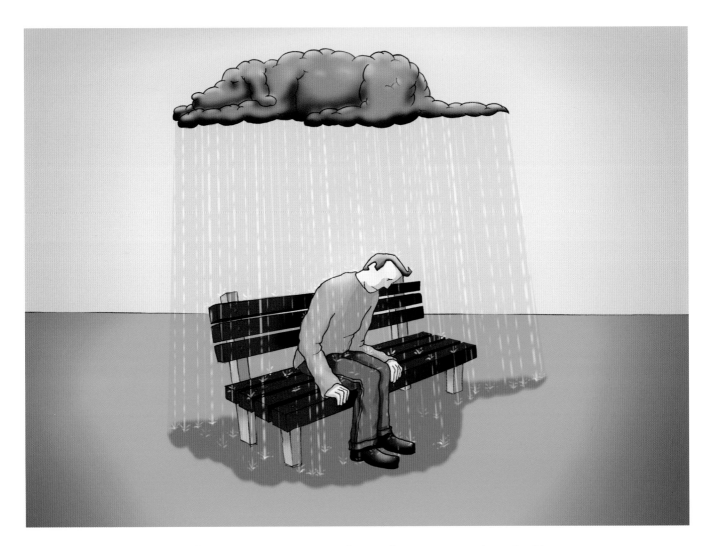

The most important thing to remember is that no matter how bad it gets ...

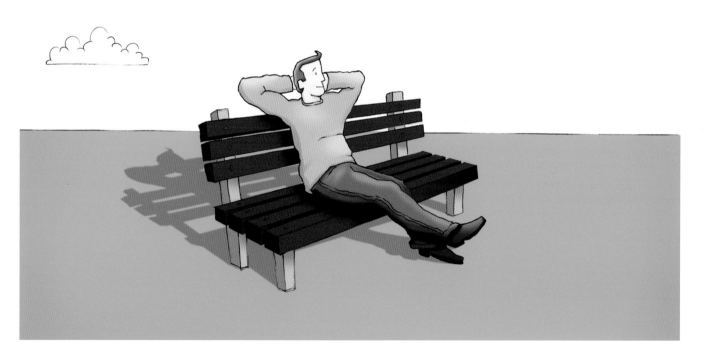

... if you take the right steps, Black Dog days can and will pass.

I wouldn't say that I am grateful for having Black Dog in my life
but what I have lost to him, I have gained in other ways.

He forced me to re-evaluate and simplify my life.

He taught me that rather than running away from problems
it's better to acknowledge and even embrace them.

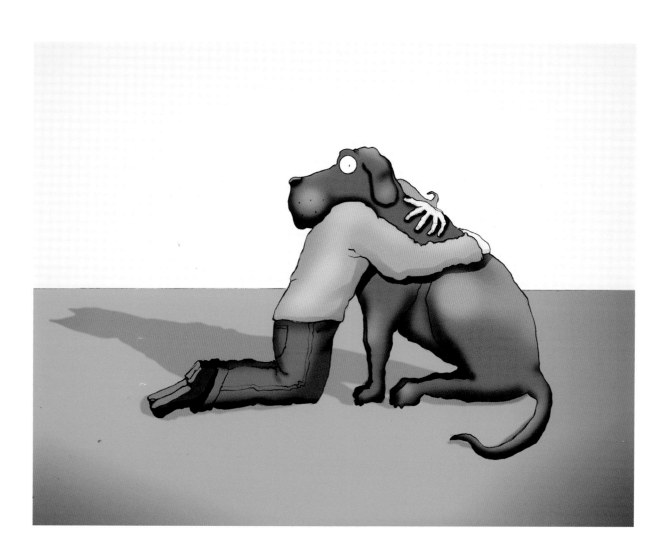

Black Dog may always be a part of my life.
But I've learnt that with patience,
humour, knowledge and discipline
even the worst Black Dog
can be made to heel.

The Beginning

ACKNOWLEDGEMENTS

I decided to create this book not so much as a self-help book but more as a visual articulation of what it is to suffer depression. I am not a psychologist, a psychiatrist nor a specialist in the field. I have merely had the unfortunate experience of suffering this terrible condition which I unaffectionately call Black Dog. I chose the Black Dog as the visual ambassador for this disease. He is an omnipresent, foul-weather fiend who permeates absolutely everything, like a drop of ink in a glass of water. My wish is that you can share this book with partners, parents, siblings, friends, even doctors and therapists. It is a visual tool that may help you articulate what you or someone you know is going through.

I would like to thank all the people who have supported me in the process of making this book. Thank you to my wonderful wife, Ainsley, who has stood by me with unconditional love, patience, humour and support. To my daughter, Abby, for bringing me so much joy and being undoubtedly the best natural antidepressant I've ever had. My dearest family and friends, who have given so much love, encouragement and support; thank you. To my literary agents, Pippa Masson, Fiona Inglis, Louise Thurtell and the staff at Curtis Brown, who believed in this project and signed me up. To Jill Wran, who introduced me to Curtis Brown. My fabulous publisher, Alex Craig, and the staff at Pan Macmillan for having the courage to buy and produce this book. To Professor Gordon Parker and the staff at the Black Dog Institute for the fantastic work they do. Gordon, your belief, support and enthusiasm made this book fly. Annie Schwebel at Mandarin Design, thank you so much for giving me a studio to work out of, and for your encouragement, creative advice and technical pearls of wisdom. To David Hutton for his support and his InDesign know how. Kathrin Ayer for taking the time to teach me how to illustrate in Photoshop. Thank you to the digital group at M&C Saatchi's for building the website: www.ihadablackdog.com. A really small, begrudging thank you to Black Dog; without you this book would have not been possible… bad dog!!!

Everyone's path to recovery is different. If you are reading this book and have a Black Dog in your life, never, ever give up the fight; Black Dog can be beaten. As Winston Churchill said, 'If you find yourself going through hell, keep going.' I wish you only peace and that you may find the quality and consistency of life that we all deserve.

Matthew Johnstone

SUGGESTED READING

Darkness Visible: A Memoir of Madness by William Styron (Vintage, 2001)

Dealing with Depression: A Common Sense Guide to Mood Disorders by Gordon Parker (Allen & Unwin, 2004)

Depression Fallout: The Impact of Depression on Couples and What You Can Do to Preserve the Bond by Anne Sheffield (HarperCollins Publishers, 2003)

Natural Prozac: Learning to Release Your Body's Own Anti-Depressants by Dr Joel Robertson with Tom Monte (HarperCollins Publishers, 1998)

The Noonday Demon: An Anatomy of Depression by Andrew Soloman (Vintage, 2002)

Overcoming Depression by Paul Gilbert (Robinson, 2000)

Undoing Depression: What Therapy Doesn't Teach You and Medication Can't Give You by Richard O'Connor, PhD (G. P. Putnam's Sons, 1999)

Wherever You Go, There You Are: Mindfulness Meditation in Everyday Life by Jon Kabat-Zinn (Piatkus Books Ltd., 2004)

HELPFUL WEBSITES

www.blackdoginstitute.org.au

www.moodgym.anu.edu.au

www.bluepages.anu.edu.au

www.undoingdepression.com

www.learningmeditation.com

www.babcp.org.uk

www.depressionalliance.org.uk

www.mind.org.uk

www.samaritans.org.uk

www.depression.org.uk

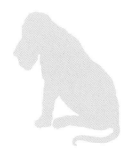